ONE IMAGINED WORD AT A TIME

Writers for Recovery

2015

WRITERS FOR RECOVERY PRESS
BARNET, VT

The following pieces have been previously published in *Epiphany*: "Hailey's Comet" and "Why I Really Went to Jail."

For more information about Writers for Recovery and how to book workshops, talks, or conference presentations, please contact Bess O'Brien at bobrien@pshift.com or go to our website at www.writersforrecovery.org

ISBN Number 9780692611517

Kingdom County Productions
949 Somers Rd. Barnet VT 05821
© 2015

Cover and interior design:
Foulkes Design

THIS ANTHOLOGY IS RESPECTFULLY DEDICATED
TO THOSE LIVING IN RECOVERY AND THOSE WHO
HAVE NOT YET FOUND THEIR WAY THERE.

Contents

I AM FROM

I Am From

by Patricia Skinner-Garvey

I am from windmills, sod houses, and hand dug wells in Wyoming,
Castles in England,
Thatched roofs in Scotland.
I am from seeds planted millennia ago by a Divine Creator.
I am from royalty and peasantry,
From kings and beggars.
I am from Portsmouth, New Hampshire on the Atlantic Ocean.
I am from Abenaki Avenue in Essex Junction, Vermont.
I am from human intellect, corn husks,
A loving fire ablaze in the heart of my mother,
And the lustful soul in the spirit of my father.
I am part of the Earth, the New England seasons,
Brutal mixes of subzero winter and tropical summers,
Lake Champlain and Mount Mansfield.
I am a woman of the Stone Age and the New Millennium
Still primitive, for our basic instincts are
The compass for survival.
I am from Yankee pride and ingenuity, strength and humor.
I am from music, love, Earth, ocean, mountains, lakes.
I am a Vermont woman.

I Am From

by Micheal Lucier

I am from small towns.
I am from 4-wheeling in the Sand Pits.
I am from long walks on logging roads
while hunting game birds with my dog, Abby.
I am from drinking coffee at my parents' store
while listening to our customers and friends
gossip about their day.
I am from drinking and partying at camp
while standing next to the bonfire telling
stories about the past week.
I am now from Northern State Correctional Facility,
paying for my mistakes.
Now I am from helping others to not make my mistakes.

I Am From

by Brandi-Lynn O'Connor

I am from combined attributes
of an egg and sperm.
The holders of each spawned
a poor decision.
I am from the child taken @ 2
to live a life with someone new.
I am from the child accepted @ 4
by an unwanting father
and an alcoholic whore.
I am from the teen whose poor
decisions led to a life of hell.
I am from the person trapped inside
Lost in confusion with nowhere to hide.
I am from the life born anew
When all pain and misery will subdue.
I am from where I'm not yet
but I know in the end
everything I'm from doesn't make
me who I am.
I am from kindness.
I am from love.
I am from freedom I hope to obtain.

I Am From

by Stan Worthley

I am from the small towns of New England, where every one knows what you had for dinner,

Where the sea was once a way of life and a badge of pride, and the resting place of lost loved ones.

I am from the back country roads we drove with no destination in mind,

Where the leaves on a cool fall day danced to the sounds of small block v8's thundering by

And the rubber left at stop signs was the only proof we were there.

I am from the place of memories both good and bad

Where I had bowed as a peasant and stood as a king,

Where the greatest of hardships showed what would become the greatest of strengths.

I know where I am from but if you ask I do not know where I'm going.

I Am From

by Pat Murray

I am from Italian streets, baked bread with a hard crust and a soft center.
I am from a breezy shore, sand and sun, endless days and nights of summer.
I am from a thousand heartaches and a hundred tears, searching for a place called home.
I am from laughter and joy and sorrow and pain and back again.
I am from a town called old fashioned and a city called wild.
I am from a long lost time forgotten in memory, too hard to remember, too painful to forget.

ADDICTION

A Morning When I Was Using

by Joshua Anderson

I would get up before she's awake
strong black coffee in the shower
  cold and to the point to save time
shaving too, avoiding eye contact
  as much as possible
leave the shower
  skin soft
    and veins popping.
Reach for my heroin hobby kit
  in the brown leather shaving bag
 I stole from my father.
Used needles,
  clean needles,
   cheap aluminum tins,
Q-tips, and tiny wax envelopes
With words like
  "Black Magic," "Reagan," and "Ambition"
stamped on them.
  I begin the ritual—
    mix the shot, find the vein,
draw back—
    push down, push off, push away.
Heroin gives me a chance, I think.
  The strength to look myself in the eyes.
I stare in the mirror and see a mask
and I adjust it
    but no matter what I do each morning
      my mask gets harder and harder
        and harder
  to breathe through.

Here's Exactly How it Happened

by Kerry Devins

I was shaking, he was smiling,

My tears, my fears

Entertaining to
His image.

He left me in the parking lot

With no shoes, without my glasses

And those broken bottles,
I couldn't catch them

And obviously, I stepped on them,
But truthfully,

The blood dripping from my toes

Led the next poor, pathetic girl

All the way home.

The Cage

by Jack Gower

My cage is built of soft clay,

Easily malleable,

Held up together by fair weather friends.

Their supports crumble at the first sign of rain.

The base is caving in, floorboards removed reveal quicksand.

How far will it pull me under this time?

The only way back up is to surrender.

To accept my plight means to finally stop

Treading and release control.

A Morning in the Middle of My Addiction

by Richard Gengras

Goddam. Stumble to the kitchen, down those friggin' stairs.
Find the ½ pint for mornings
Puke
Drink water.
Get sorta right, put on pants, shirt
It's 7:45.

Walk to the Center, get a pint at 8:00
And start walking home, drinking, in public.
No shame, no cares.

All of Hartford going to work.
Shit.
I gotta get to work—not till 10:00.
Have a drink boys-your loving bride awaits you!

Yeah-right, she awaits something.

Fuck, I'm tired. Get some blow on the way in.

I wish I was back on heroin.

Gotta puke again.

Mom calls, says I'm drinking again.
How does she know?

I haven't talked to anyone today.

Hailey's Comet

Kevin Fuller

I was there when you were born. A new man had to be sworn. Got hurt, my head was torn. Got mad wouldn't eat your corn. Tough guy turned to Jello, being dad made me mellow. That's when people saw me, the good fellow. Missed your birthdays turned me yellow. When you are gone my mind is a hearse. It's like a neverending curse. I am stuck, stuck in reverse. That's when I met the demon, drugs, bad excuses, but miss our bear hugs. In your pictures you're getting older. I fear with age I will get a cold shoulder. Poison minded thoughts corrupt. Sobriety halted, started abrupt. Out there I felt like your hero. In here I am a minus one to zero. Family badly ashamed. Still this wild heart couldn't be tamed. It's me, everyone I blamed to the burnt bridges badly maimed. I haven't seen you since eight or nine but still pretended everything was fine. Cowboy up, stop the whine. You still have plenty, plenty of time. The clock is still ticking so stay out the grime. I have to think the thoughts of good choices. No need to listen, others' voices. I think of you every day, you probably wonder when I am here to stay. You're on the top shelf. To get there I have to work on myself. Should be a given, shouldn't hard but it's a trap. Slicked with lard. It starts by feeling sad, I cry, then I get mad. To feel better I then get high, some relief I blow out a sigh. It changes me, that I can't deny. Like a wolf, howl at the moon. Don't wake up until the afternoon. I sit here all alone. It's impossible, the way cannot be shown. Blinded by all the hate. I wonder if this is it, my fate. Please help me on this quest. I swear on Hailey's comet, my behavior is at its best.

There Are Things That Keep Him Awake in the Night

by Nick Piliero

His head strikes the pillow, but comfort is not there
His brain is racing, but goes nowhere
The film of his day, the movie of his life
They all seem to come to him dead in the night
Things that were done and things that were not
They all line up, put his stomach in a knot
Sleep will not come as he tosses and turns
Thinking has become the monster that takes over his brain
Oh, how he hates those who easily lie down and fall to sleep

This is Something I Wanted to Tell You

by Robert Cote

Look through the eyes of the ones who love you. Watch with us as we watch you disintegrate. When you look through my eyes, do you see what I see? The hollow eyes of a doped-up prom queen. The staggered steps of someone we look up to. When we look through the memories we created, do you see the graceful moves as you dance with me? How about the fogless sparkle in your eyes when you put on that ring?

Waking Up in Addiction

by Nancy Bassett

Oh wow, what time is it? It's kind of dark out there. Crap, it's pouring—I can hear it on the roof & splatting against the windows.

I need coffee... OK, first things first. I sit up... I look over next to me... Is Wayne awake? Yes!! Time to get high... Come on Wayne, move it—hurry up—can I go first this morning?
Pleeeze?

I sit up and grab the little green quilted bag stored in the drawer next to my side of the bed. After Wayne sits up & reaches over to turn up the lamp, I hand the bag to him. He unzips it & starts laying everything out.

OK, I'll start the coffee while you're fixing it. Have we got enough for the day? No? Shit, we're gonna have to go to Springfield—do we have the money we need? Yes? Awesome!
Now hurry up, come on, hurry up!

Oh man, we were going to spend the day with our kid, it's Matt's day off. We're going to have to tell him some story—something... that we can't hang out with him today. We were going to drive up to camp—shit, shit, shit!!!! Well, we'll call him in a little while...

OK, it's ready? I fix the tie, hold out my arm & feel the prick. Ahhhh, better now... I close my eyes for a minute & feel the wet, cold swipe of the sharp smelling rubbing alcohol in the crook of my arm.

My day has begun... I'm good for a while...

Why I Really Went to Jail

by Gavin Howley

Since I am generally extremely concerned about how people perceive me, and worried that they may not have the complete picture of my amazing depth and complex personality, with like, real issues and stuff, you know, such a fascinating person that all I think about is myself and only those events going on that have a direct impact on me, I agonize over appearance and every spoken utterance, usually agonizing over making myself look like I don't care about any of that, again, because I'm so deep, man. And if I'm around a woman I don't know too well, but whose proximity increases my heart rate out of fear she might not like me, all this nonsense is of course multiplied by infinity. I've been in this state yet again recently, which seems to be a pattern I like to repeat. I'm just dying to demonstrate to her that I'm a person worth being interested in, but how do I do this? Trying to be funny seems to be my default mode, and that includes trying way, way too hard. To the point where it is obvious that I spent a scary amount of time preparing whatever it is, a thing or a wacky personal anecdote, anything. But ever since a friend called me flaky, years and years ago, I have this desperate need to show that I've been through things, dealt with pain and bad things, and consequently have all these deep emotions and shit that other people might just not get. Yeah it's a tiring way to live life and the payoff, if you will, for all this anxiety and time spent mostly doing and saying nothing because that would involve decisions has been basically zero.

What does this have to do with jail? Reasonable question. Just about all of the pain and bad experiences I've racked up happened simply through being an addict, a pretty bad one, I'd say. So lately I wonder a lot about using any of that as a way to show normal people why I'm interesting and stuff. Since over the years the only constant life events and growth has been in the field of drinking a lot and devouring powders and pills, that is, or feels like, the major part of who I am. So of course I try to figure out how to let new people know this in a way that makes me look good somehow. And adding the year in jail as the latest accomplishment only makes my brain try to spin that in a way that shows I like, have a badass side or something. Since jail in Swanton, Vermont is as rough as it gets.

The question of exactly how I ended up there probably would come up. At first I like to say just "drugs" or "heroin" or "drug stuff." Never alcohol, and especially not DUIs. There's nothing cool at all about DUIs. The thing is I got the first two through textbook alcoholic drinking. I may as well have just followed an instruction manual. Probation, CRASH, all that stuff. It is true that DUI 3 had nothing to do with alcohol, and yes I had started heroin by then, and shooting everything, and all the cool stuff like that, but it just came down to driving a car while all fucked up, and getting caught, again.

The sentence was 1-3 years but I could stay out if I was sober and completed a lot of time in programs and groups. At the time I hated my PO but he really did try to keep me out and have a chance to lead some sort of life. But all I wanted to do was steal drugs from sharps containers in the exam rooms at my job at the Community Health Center. Prying the lid off, dumping everything on the floor and pawing at the pile of needles for disposed pills. Hoping no one would come in. Then a doctor left a box of fentanyl patches on a desk one day. That was a no-brainer. Also getting caught was a no-brainer for the police. I was a known addict on supervision at the time and only one of a few people who could have possibly taken them. So with that, I got put in the car and driven up to Swanton.

They even tried to get me out of jail and do some more programs and another rehab. I, apparently, was determined to "keep coming back," just not exactly in the AA manner. The booking officers shook their heads the three times I left and then returned within a month. I had no way to get alcohol and drugs anymore but still needed to fuck up my brain. I remembered hearing in a rehab that teenagers were getting high on Dust-Off, the canned air for electronics. Anything was something I would try by then, and Kmart and Radio Shack were close. Not good. That stuff is bad, bad news. I would stand in front of a mirror with it and feel outside myself and like I was staring at someone I did not recognize. I thought I left the planet, I thought I was a ghost, I was positive I was in an alternate dimension. It just about always ended in a blackout and collapsing wherever I happened to be. You can basically feel the brain cells dying. So naturally I had to have it constantly.

Within probably less than two weeks I got myself banned and issued no trespass orders from any CCTA bus, the downtown mall, the YMCA, any public park, and any UVM property. My life was getting up, walking to Kmart and standing by the door until they opened at eight. I'd get let in with my big down jacket on, fill it up with all the cans I could, and walk out. I have no idea how I avoided arrest with that. It wasn't subtle. Then I'd find an indoor place, since it was winter, and suck down cans until I blacked out. Sometimes I woke up, kept going, and blacked out somewhere else and sometimes I awoke in the ER. They released me from the ER once without removing any cans from my backpack, and I was back in 20 minutes, not even making it out of the building. Someone found me in the lobby bathroom. One time the collapsing part was in the street on Shelburne Road. I got delusional, paranoid, forgot who I was, and just plain hallucinated stuff. The places I could legally enter in the winter were getting slim so a bus shelter or the woods had to do. Suffice to say these activities somehow kept bringing me back to AB or I unit at Northwestern State Correctional Facility. The last time they let me out on supervision, I returned in less than 24 hours after bringing the stuff to my check-in at the Phoenix House.

So this is the recent history that I want to misguidedly twist into a reason to be likable. My fear of not being liked and rejection or god forbid someone having a not-positive thought still runs the show a good percentage of the time, so I get caught up in constant self-centered thinking mode, feeling that I need to be liked by others in order for me to feel ok with myself. And it's especially agonizing when wanting a particular woman to think I'm likable. Some of the stuff I've done in just the year since getting out and a job at a building that doesn't only contain men is super cringe-worthy. "Desperate flirting" I'd call it. No wonder people are maybe not backing away, but giving me a little space. I'm so self-centered that I cannot even attempt fictional writing or creating characters that are not just myself. I don't think I could write about a different personality and have it be believable. It would be a shallow movie-poster person. It's like my mind just cannot grasp the concept of other thoughts besides my own. I need to stay aware of this. The next time I consider using jail to appear a certain way to someone I need to just think about saying: "I spent a year in jail for huffing. That's right, I huff things. I'm a huffer. A bad one. Huffer Seeks Soulmate." Well, enough. That's a sad world to get lost in.

The Real Me

by Naibar Kahz

Insecure,
Think I'm smart, but not for sure,
Really scared of kissing her.

Fearful, fearful little boy,
Angry cuz you stole my toy.

Racing thoughts, such a mess,
Non-stop anxiety,
Read the Torah to impress,
But no real sense of piety,
I'll never fit in this society.

Smallest kid on the playground,
Angry parents, often frowned.

The coolest kid,
I want to be,
Won't let you know the real me
Happy, fun—don't give a fuck—
That's what I want you to see.

Friends say I own
my sexuality.
Delusion sewn
by a fallacy.

Put up a front; I love that self,
But guilty about my parents wealth,
Forced to make a joke of my mental health,
Take a look at my trophy shelf,
But alone at home, I want to kill myself.

So ashamed/of my past,
Façade of perfection will never last,
Give me the bong, one more blast,
To leave the club, I'm always last.

I pretend I'm an intellectual,
4 yrs.—16 credits—I'm just ineffectual,
I'm only good at being sexual.

Debate, debate, debate, debate...
Fearful and lonely. Is this my fate?

Combating shame,
A war in my head,
Battling pain,
Wish I were dead.

Can't pull the trigger.
Instead, go figure:
In-no-cent casualties
Ian! Ian! Call us please...

You say I'm so hot
I say not
"So pensitive"
Just sensitive

"So mature and put together"
Could rock my ego with a feather
Bipolar thoughts like a ball on a tether
Can't stop this lightning, dark, stormy weather.

Call it cognitive dissonance
Emotionally sober, haven't been since...
Caron. Now, I'm back again
Caring? How? Instead of sin?

I have a choice
I hear God's voice
Main Caron to bane Caron
I've come full circle
Pain-bearing to sane sharing
I wanna be a whole circle

Siege the wall of defense
Return to my sense
I wanna be...
The real me.
Caron. Now, I'm back again
Caring? How? Instead of sin?

I have a choice
I hear God's voice
Main Caron to bane Caron
I've come full circle
Pain-bearing to sane sharing
I wanna be a whole circle

Siege the wall of defense
Return to my sense
I wanna be...
The real me.

The Cage of My Depression

by Sarah Ferland

Isolation...
Silence...
Nothing but my own thoughts to occupy me.

Everyone is gone;
I am just left here,
Forgotten...

The voices come and go,
Telling me my anxieties
Then leaving me alone.

"Why did you even bother to get up today?"

"Don't speak,
You know no one wants to hear you!"

"I wonder what would happen
If we walked into traffic...
Looks fun!"

"Blood is the only release you will get;
So pick,
Scratch,
Go ahead and bring a knife to the party!"

"Time to go to bed
Hopefully you won't wake up again..."

My Drinking Days

by Connie Perry

I would go to the bar, get drunk
Someone would pick me up.

I have gone to dead-end roads
To have sex.

Not caring if I made it back.

I would come to.
Not knowing where I was or who the other person was.

I did not catch a sex disease.

Thank you for my life.

I did not care.

I would not be missed.

I was a nobody out there.

Those were my drinking days.

The Things That Keep Him Awake At Night

by Kaleb Kelly

These are the things that keep him awake at night. Terror, horror, and depression. Nothing to do with his lack of sleep. He retires to bed, but with thoughts that seem like a child who has ingested a god-awful amount of caffeine. It's the simple things he lies awake at night pondering. They say try and breathe in this pattern or try to bore yourself with a simple question. Still, he overthinks things. He tries to empty his mind but it seems as he rids himself of one issue, that they multiply endlessly. Where does it end? How? He seeks help from yoga, meditation, and other silly methods, but still to no avail. Maybe he is cursed to have the wandering mind, like a ghost doomed to wander until he has finished his business.

RECOVERY

Why I Write for My Recovery

by John Gower

Remember when you were very young lying alone in a field or park and the clouds overhead somehow resonated in an idle sort of way with images and stories deep within your soul? Of course it was silly, but it still mattered, and mattered deeply. Writing for recovery is connecting with that very important silliness. Before we learned how not to be, it never occurred to us that we weren't wonderful. Writing for recovery gives us play and gives us heart. It suspends in midair the possibility of what might happen next. This unleashing of uncertainty moves us across the high wire, where balance only comes from moving the story along. One word followed by the next, we move our wonderful life forward while the crowd looks on in awe, and balance comes not by looking down or back, but from imagining where you're going next. Writing for recovery is recovering your balance. It is moving your life forward, one imagined word at a time.

A Morning Clean and Sober

by Anonymous

"I like it here," I explain. I want him to understand why I am absolutely motionless.

Overnight, the bed became softer and warmer. The colors in the room are playing very nicely together; I'm noticing how much I love these curtains. They're just so right.

I can hear him open the cupboard, grab a cup, pour coffee. He gives a Splenda packet a few taps, his coffee a stir, the spoon lands on the side of the sink. I'm still unwilling to budge. I find the covers over my head, and bliss.

Dear Addiction

by Caitlin Ferland

This is what you told me, no matter the time, no matter the day, no matter what was going on in life, all the time:

If 2 feels good, 10 is much better.
How can you do anything without me by your side?
How much have you got? You know what happens if you run out.
You already fucked up today, might as well keep going.
Make sure you don't feel. There's too much pain to face.
You look OK; at least you have me.
They won't understand. They don't know what you've gone through or the things that   you've done.
At least you haven't done that yet. You're not that bad.
Whatever he wants, just give it to him. It'll help you forget.
Just tell them what they want to hear. We can figure it out later.
Don't ignore me. I'm not going away.
You don't deserve a good life; look at you now.

But the truth is:

I am powerless over you, without God to help me.
I am worth sobriety, no matter what you say.
Perfection is not possible, but progress feels good.
My best effort is good enough.
It is not OK to neglect my kids
Not OK to steal
Not OK to lie
Not OK to live in my head and listen to you
No OK to abuse my body
Not OK to not pray
Not OK to skip meetings
Not OK to not talk to my sponsor
Not OK to have any mind or mood altering substance in my body.
It is OK to be good to myself.
It is OK to help others with this disease; it is necessary to do so to stay sober.

You lie to me always, hurt me when you can,
Take my job, my home, my kids, and will take
My life if I don't recover. You take my
Worth, my love, my everything.
I am done with you and all of your lies.
Today God is keeping me sober and restoring my life.
Today my higher power is keeping me sober
And the truth is all I want.

What I Want My Mother to Know

by Bob Purvis

My addiction is not your fault—any more than Dad's alcoholism was your fault. It's a disease that, once churning along at its chosen and ever-accelerating speed, will fuel one bad choice after another, ultimately leading me to bend or break every relationship that is important to me—to fracture the life I had built into a million pieces.

But here's another thing you need to know about my addiction: whatever its source or influences, I am accountable for every bad choice that I made, and I am responsible for making the consequences of those choices right.

You have often said you are proud of what I have accomplished during my life in recovery.

But those accomplishments were only possible because I came to accept my addiction as something that is a part of me, that I must live with and work through every day.

So whether or not I deserve the credit you give me, I will accept it on one condition: that you must let me own my addiction. This is what you need to know.

I'll Never Forget That Day

By John Preterotti

I'll never forget that day
That I made my father proud,
Playing baseball like him.

I'll never forget that day
Driving my bike far from
Home, free and happy on
A sunny day.

I'll never forget that day
My best friend passed away.

I'll never forget that day
That I received my
Business license at age 19,
Copper Valley Roofing.

I'll never forget that day
I met my future
Wife and now
Mother of my children.

I'll never forget that day
My princess, my daughter,
Was born.

I'll never forget that day
Daddy's little boy
Was brought into this world.

I'll never forget the day
I walk away from the bad
And walk that straight line
For myself and my children.
That day is here.
I will not forget this day.

This Is What I Wanted to Tell You

by George Thomas

So, Bingo, this is what I wanted to tell you. I've noticed that you rarely hang with friends and you often avoid calling me back.

Others have reported the same runaround. (Sue) Your oboe practice sessions have gotten much shorter. (Wayne) You burn with an unfixated anger that doesn't die away. Worry pulls your
face like a downward dog.

Wanna share what's happening? You were there for me before I got into the rooms. I'm listening.

I Forgive Myself for That Time When...

by Kristen L. Lafond

I Forgive Myself for That Time When...

I held in what I was feeling
I held it in because
I didn't want to show you
I have trouble forgiving myself
because I keep forgetting
that I am only human
I am only one person
I cannot do it all
Sometimes I can't do anything

I'm at a loss
I don't know what to say
I forgive myself
for that time when...
for every time when.

I forgive you
   I forgive you
      I forgive you

I say, as I stand
in front of the mirror
Then I smile
as I walk away
because I've finally
forgiven myself for that time when...

Sobriety Stew

by Kurtis Thompson

1 tender and loving Mom
1 already seasoned old school Stepfather
1 Heavenly spirited big sister (for inspiration)
2 20 lb. cats (extra cuddly and playful)
3 cups of therapy
1 cup going back to school to become a teacher
2 tbsp. writing and reading every day
2 tbsp. music (the cosmic dance of the soul)
2 tbsp. laughter

Season liberally with forgiveness, patience, understanding and love.
Stir gently and often.
Allow to simmer One Day at a Time.

When Someone I Know is Using

by Brent Edward Farrell

Part of me feels the ache of desire
For loves lost,
For dreams never fulfilled.
Then comes the pain of remembering,
The crushing reality of what the outcome inevitably becomes...
Despair.
The fleeting joy, the serendipitous smile
The void of my emptiness registering in their face
Thankful it isn't me anymore,
On the Ferris wheel gone haywire.
Thankful the truth has been crawled through,
And the light shines... All around.

Peace.

What I Have Recovered

by Joseph Scalzo

I only recovered a part of my life that I lost so long ago.
I've found family that were lost.

I only recovered a part of me that is for life.

I'm always going to have that thought of ending my life,

but I've put that on hold and realized my fears, my past, my now.
I have only truly just started my recovery because of all I tried to hide away.

Trying to pull myself into the light instead of living in the dark.

Recipe for Support
by Jenn Dilworth

2 cups patience
2 cups comfort
5 bushels love
3 cups caring
3 cups understanding
5 cups listening
3 cups faith
2 cups a shoulder to cry on
1/2 cup compassion
1/2 cup honesty
2 cups prayer

Shift and mix the ingredients together
and you have a support person.

What I Have Recovered

by Ryan J. Smith

I'm still in the process of losing.
Nothing has yet been recovered.
One day I woke up and it was all gone.
Everything I knew and loved was mine no more.
The woman of my dreams called the police.
I was told I no longer had a place to call home.
I couldn't even say goodbye to my children.
My furniture, TVs, silverware, dishes,
even my washer & dyer were gone forever.
I thought I still had my freedom,
but that was taken, too.
I was ready to give up,
but I refuse to give in.
Every day I wake up and tell myself
"Today is the day my life begins."

The Person Who is my Secret Weapon

by Matt Adams

The person who is my secret weapon in staying sober is my son, Ashton. Ashton was born on February 24th of this year. He's just four months old and is the biggest inspiration in my life to becoming fully sober. I spend almost all of every day with Ashton because he's an amazing blessing. He's the most beautiful person, and to not be sober around him would just be a huge disappointment. It's like he is so new to the world and as pure as can be, so why be high around him and ruin it?

Spending time with Ashton has its own type of euphoria, where you always have a smile, whether he's being playful, sleeping, upset, or even sad. I couldn't imagine being here today without Ashton in my life. I'd either be down the street getting high or overdosed and dead. I love Ashton and I am so grateful and appreciative that I have him in my life. Ashton will always be my secret weapon in recovery, and in anything else I have to deal with for the rest of my life.
I love you, Ashton.

A Morning Clean and Sober

by Noah Lowry

I wake up to my phone ringing, it's my mother calling me on the first of the month to say *rabbit rabbit*. We joke for a sec and then get off the phone. Before I do anything I stop and say a prayer and thank God for waking me up. I walk into the bathroom not even thinking about the mirror and proceed to take a shower and brush my teeth. I go into the kitchen and start making my usual breakfast, eggs, sausage, and onion and turn on SportsCenter so I can get my much-needed sports news. I sit in my living room eating my breakfast as well, as my cat eats right beside me, we look at each other as if we are saying 'Today is gonna be a good day.' I get up, go outside feeling nothing but happiness and thank the Lord for a beautiful day and then I say to myself, 'Another day sober,' and continue with my day.

I Win

by Angala Devoid

The moment I felt you tickle my throat. The moment I felt the warmth of your touch run through my body, I knew I was hooked. I ached for you, I cried for you, I dreamed about you until you were in my arms once more.

When I put you to my lips the passion was so overwhelming I was willing to die for you to go to jail for you to lose my kids for you to lose the respect of family, friends, my community for you. But most of all I was willing to lose myself for you. You had ahold of me so tight as you were laughing at me the whole time until one day I got honest and said no more I looked up and yelled Higher power I do not believe in you right now but I need help here I'm not ready to die!

So I learned to fight this battle of the bottle that I thought in my mind was my best friend, my lover, my everything one day at a time I know I'm a winner and not a prisoner of that bottle I held in my arms like a baby all the time.

FREEWRITE

Technically, He Had Never Done This Before

by Anonymous

Technically, he had never done this before, but how hard could it be?

You like a girl who lives in Colorado. She's invited you to stay with her.

You bartend. I'm pretty sure there are bars everywhere.

You've been saying you are going to get out of NJ since high school. Do you really want to be one of those people who can't live anywhere else because you're afraid you won't know how to make a bagel?

Step 1- The decision to leave.

Step 2- Put stuff in car.

Step 3- Look at a map; find Colorado.

Step 4- "Oh, it's over there."

Step 5- Go there.

As so began a new life. I was only 22 at the time. I've had many unique experiences, learned so much. But perhaps the most important thing I've learned is that it's true; nobody knows how to make a bagel. Jesus Christ, you can't just put a hole in a piece of bread and call it a bagel, that's fucking bullshit.

That Warm Day

by Brandy Hunt

The fact was that all that warm weather and sunshine was making her feel just awful. The day had been very hot and muggy, with no sign of letting up any time soon. This didn't bother Esme, though, because these days turned into the best kind of nights. The kind perfect for long walks in the woods behind her house. The only problem was what to do until nightfall. When she was young, this wouldn't have been a problem. Esme could close her eyes and just let her imagination run wild. Now at the age of 22 she had lost that part of her and it wasn't likely to return. So, without one more thought about it, she went right outside into that awful heat that made her feel equally as awful—and she kept walking until she got to the woods where she had played all her life.

She walked past the little brook at the entrance to the pathway and continued to walk until she hit the old quarry hole where her parents had taken her since an early age. Slowly, she took off all her clothing until she was completely nude and jumped off the ledge into the deep quarry. Just like that, Esme felt like a kid again, like no time had passed at all. Esme was young again.

My Father's Hands

by Leslie Bonette

My father wasn't like Mr. Wonson,
With his soft, flabby lips
And protruding belly.

My father was tall and lean and handsome
And looked like he could be somebody famous
"Like he stepped out of a bandbox," my mother said
Only I didn't know anything about bandboxes.

He had the hands of an artist
Strong and gentle
I'd watch them
When he drew cartoons for me.

My father wasn't like Mr. Wonson
Who used to pull the drapes
And try to kiss me.

My father bought me jewelry and fancy dresses
Took me to dinner and dancing.
He'd put my tiny feet on his and we'd whirl across the floor
Me, drunk on his cologne, he on his martinis.

My father wasn't like Mr. Lindars
Who asked the little girls into his garage
And had them pull their pants down.

My father picked me up every Sunday
And we'd go visiting
I'd sit quietly in my scratchy dress
While the grown ups laughed and ate.

He'd carry me drowsy to the car
We'd soar down silent parkways
In the blackness he'd pull me close.

My father's hands didn't seem like an artist's then and
I wished he'd leave them on the steering wheel
And me on my side of the car.

My father wasn't like Mr. Sarlin
The kind teacher who saw trouble in my eyes
And shed a tear when he read a poem I wrote.

My father cried when he had too much to drink.
He told me he didn't know how to be a father
And I believed him.

Who was this stinking man
Who had the neighbors keep watch on me?
Always needing to know where I was,
He said he'd show me just who was boss.

My father would have men with axe handles
Follow me and call my name
And then disappear.

These nameless, faceless men always seemed to know
Just where I'd be and
Just what jewelry I'd be wearing.
I couldn't hide from my father's hands.

No, my father wasn't like Mr. Wonson
Who would pull the drapes and try to kiss me
Or Mr. Lindars hiding in his garage.

My father was a silent, insidious stalker
Who seduced the little girl who thought he was God.

Three Openings

by Tavid Bingham

Even behind a door, he felt a glare. An all-seeing eye of judgment. The windows could be shut and the shades drawn, and still the fear of revealing failure would be there. If they didn't know what he was up to, there in that little room in the dark, they were sure to realize it when he came out. The way his face sagged, or flushed. He had so many tells. Over time he'd grown accustomed to making these tells. Always with the knowledge that someone would be watching. It was harder and then easier and then harder again to fool the watchers. But if he could keep the fooling easier, he'd be comfortable.

He woke up in bed alone. The person who should have been there with him wasn't. That was the first thing he noticed. The second thing he noticed was the throbbing pressure hanging onto the insides of his skull. Pulling them in with the pressure of a star about to collapse in on itself. He rolled over and breathed heavily, checking to make sure she wasn't just on the other side. Of course not. She wouldn't be there. They always slept on the same sides of the bed. He on the right and she on the left. Unless of course they were in a new place. A hotel, or a friend or relative's, perhaps away on a trip. Wait, that's where he was. In a hotel room, but not his, not theirs. The pressure in his head sharpened and dulled cyclically. What had happened? Where was Ann? Why was he there, alone?

They had not even known she was missing. She often spent much of most nights up in her room, as mother would say, doing "god knows what." And she didn't move around very much, so there wasn't much in the way of floorboard creaks or murmurs to remind those of us downstairs that she was there. The fans twirled while mother did her knitting and father read the newspaper, smoking his pipe and hardly blinking. At one point, mother had said, "I've made that appointment for her to see the doctor next month. They couldn't get her in sooner." Father grunted, approvingly, but not many would know that by his tone. Later in the evening when that knock came at the door, father looked up from his paper. "Who could that be?"

In There

by Dianne Richardson

In there
inside the elbow
I see
the old woman
the wrinkled skin
loose & sagging.

Out there,
in the outstretched arm,
I see
the young woman,
full of vitality, strength,
and courage.

Between the two
is me.

Avian April

by Carol Van Etten

A dozen black birds swoop up into the sky as I gaze upwards at the clouds
Upon disembarking from my trusty old Ford Focus at Woodridge Rehab.
The air is cool, and sprinkled with rain drops during this chilly April.
The sudden movement of the flock makes me stop in awe at the beauty
And serenity of the scene, where the fluttering wings momentarily persist.
The sound dissipates as the birds move beyond the nearby building.
From within, through a large bay window, a friend witnesses
The awesome activity of the flock in flight from the nearby stark tree branches.
To observe and be observed is miraculous this fine spring day in April!
Ever present as well are a shower of snowflakes—not an uncommon sight.
Soon, tiny mint leaves will appear as buds and then eventually be transformed.
The birds had so recently perched on the tree before departing in haste.
The symmetry of the motion of the group appears effortless yet beautiful –
A natural event that occurs with a nonchalance to be appreciated by all!

In the Beginning, All I Wanted Was a Normal Life

by Jim Dines

In the beginning, all I wanted was a normal life, then I found out what normal was as far as most people were concerned. I wasn't sure I could have it, but I was certain that whatever I wanted out of life, normal wasn't it.

Looking back, I was a sort of budding Buckminster Fuller; I cast out everything I was taught. Everything I was told was true. Everything I once thought I knew, I now knew that I never knew. From that moment forward every idea and ideal I held in my mind, in my heart, was mine, though I'd be equally happy if you shared it, too.

The truth is I didn't succeed in casting out my ill preconceptions, but I tried, harder than most, I feel.

I did succeed, though. I succeeded in redefining success in my mind to a state that is always attainable.

Even when broke, homeless, alone, that is a feeling, I think, that most have never known.

Ode to the Mail Carrier

by Don Henry

You come every day except Sunday, thank you.
You leave those horrific bills and flyers from Kinney Drugs, those, you may keep.
Waiting for a check, which never seems to come. It's needed to pay my bills.
I honor you for delivering in snow, sleet and freezing rain.
I appreciate you also taking my outgoing mail, my paid bills, Christmas cards, RSVP's
and invites to weddings and social events.
Receiving mail addressed to my neighbor, a mistake, however an open invitation to
meet someone unknown and possibly a new friend.
You bring joy and sorrow, good news and bad, but without you, my daily chore of
getting the mail would no longer be something that I look forward to every day.
Thank you.

Contributors

MATT ADAMS is a writer from the Barre Writers for Recovery Workshop.

JOSHUA ANDERSON was born and raised in Underhill Center, Vermont. He graduated from Emerson College in Boston and did graduate studies in political science at UMass Amherst. He lives in Burlington, Vermont with his beautiful wife Shanon and their black labs Rosie and Trooper.

NANCY BASSETT returned to the Northeast Kingdom in 2002, after 16 months of Federal Bureau of Prisons supervision in CT & MA. She worked as a coordinator at the Kingdom Recovery Center in St. Johnsbury, VT for 10 ½ years. She is now a recovery coach, facilitator of a nurturing parenting group, and recovery advocate.

TAVID BINGHAM was born in Philadelphia but grew up in northern Vermont. Professional credits include landscaper, campaign field manager, cab driver, snow reporter, sunflower seed peddler and winter vacation promoter. When he's not going in hundred different directions he's working on writing, and understanding that drinking and use don't help him to be a better writer.

LESLIE BONETTE began writing when she was in about 5th or 6th grade; at least anything that was worth reading. Taking a writing class with Jim Ellefson at Champlain College some years ago inspired her to continue. Leslie loves Writers for Recovery because we care about and get encouragement from each other.

ROBERT COTE is a writer from the Caledonia Writers for Recovery Workshop

KERRY DEVINS is a writer from the Burlington Writers for Recovery Workshop.

ANGALA DEVOID has been in recovery for 12 1/2 years.
She drank to forget yesterdays and hide her feelings, to be liked and accepted. Once she admitted she was an alcoholic her life changed, one day at a time. She is a great mother, sister, daughter, friend, and member of her community today.

JENN DILWORTH is a writer from the Barre Writers for Recovery Workshop.

JIM DINES is a writer from the Burlington Writers for Recovery Workshop.

BRENT EDWARD FARRELL is a native Vermonter, who moved back to experience sobriety after many years in California. He has been active in the Burlington community since arriving here in 2014. He worked at the Low Barrier Shelter with CVOEO in the winter of 2014/15. Presently he works with a consignment clothing store in Burlington getting quality clothes to those in need free of charge.

CAITLIN FERLAND is a recovering alcoholic/addict. She has found a new way to heal through her writing. She has been blessed with the gift of sobriety and writing is one of many joys she has found.

SARAH FERLAND struggled throughout her childhood with depression and anxiety. She found solace in literature and visual art. She currently writes short stories for blogs, sometimes accompanied by her own digital artwork. Sarah is studying software engineering at Vermont Technical College.

KEVIN FULLER was born and raised in Newbury, Vermont. A writer and visual artist, he enjoys bass fishing and working on and driving high performance cars. "Hailey's Comet," was written in "the hole" while Kevin was in the custody of the Vermont Department of Corrections.

PATRICIA SKINNER-GARVEY was born in Portsmouth, NH in 1952, and has been a resident of Vermont since 1954. She's a graduate of Essex Junction High School and the University of Vermont. Patty is the extremely proud mother of three grown children, Dr. Sean M. Garvey, Master Case Thomas Garvey, and Ms. Greta Brooke Garvey.

RICHARD GENGRAS moved to Vermont with his family in the late 1980s, and moved from Killington to Danville in the late 90s. He is a chef and a singer and songwriter.

Embarrassingly, **JACK GOWER** was born and raised in Florida but moved to Vermont a year and a half ago. Try not to hold that against him; we think he means well. He spends most of his time these days trying to be funny in the form of writing.

JOHN GOWER lives in Burlington, VT in a furnished room. He is employed as a drug and alcohol counselor and has been previously published in Epiphany literary magazine. John sometimes leaves his writing in Laundromats for others to enjoy.

DON HENRY was born in Montpelier, VT and in 1972 moved to Barre, where he currently resides. He became involved with Writers for Recovery to explore his writing ability and form fellowships with others in recovery. The workshop has been important in helping him understand his alcoholism, which is important to his recovery.

GAVIN HOWLEY (1973-present) is most experienced in the field of using alcohol and drugs to avoid life. After a one-year stint in jail, he decided it was time to work on accepting life as it comes, warts and all, putting himself out there as far as music and writing is concerned, and trying to worry less about what people may be thinking about him.

BRANDY HUNT is a writer from the Barre Writers for Recovery Workshop.

NAIBAR KAHZ is the pen name of Ian Robert Hemley, a writer, slam poet, non-traditional student and political communications consultant. Now a recovered addict, Ian enjoys hiking, tennis, skiing, and slam poetry. He works in communications at Rights and Democracy, a political non-profit in the Old North End of Burlington, Vermont.

KALEB KELLY is a writer from the Caledonia Writers for Recovery Workshop.

KRISTEN L. LAFOND is Assistant Director of the Turning Point Center of Central Vermont.

NOAH LOWRY is a writer from the Barre Writers for Recovery Workshop.

MICHEAL LUCIER was born and raised in Vermont's Northeast Kingdom, where he played, hunted in the woods, and attended North Country Union High School. After a long struggle with drugs and alcohol, he ended up in jail, where he is finishing an eight-year sentence. His goal is to get a college education and teach others not to follow in his footsteps.

PAT MURRAY was born in Philadelphia, PA and moved to Barre, Vermont in 2009 with her partner to pursue their dream of a life together in Vermont. Pat has been sober over 3 years and became involved with Writers for Recovery to stay connected with others in recovery and pursue a dream of someday writing a book.

BRANDI-LYNN O'CONNOR is a writer from the Newport Writers for Recovery Workshop.

CONNIE PERRY has been sober for 11 1/2 years. Thanks to this, she has her family back.

NICK PILIERO is a self-taught artist whose career came to him in a vision in a near death experience. He has sold paintings all over the world, but writing is new to him. Nick grew up in the Bronx, New York City, and has lived in Vt. for 22 years. Nick has 21 years in recovery and two sons that he had late in life, at ages 54 and 56.

JOHN PRETEROTTI was raised mostly in Western Massachusetts and Connecticut. He is a father of two, a contractor, and a lover of sports, hunting, and living life to the fullest. He is serving a sentence for possession at the Northern State Correctional in Newport Vermont and practicing sobriety.

BOB PURVIS is Director of the Turning Point Center of Central Vermont.

DIANNE RICHARDSON has lived in Montpelier, Vermont most of her 61 years. She loves all the arts. She is especially drawn to butterflies, animals, poetry, drawing, music, yoga, spirituality and all open-hearted expressions. Wellness and recovery, especially through the arts, is also a major focus of her life.

JOSEPH SCALZO is a writer from the Newport Writers for Recovery Workshop.

RYAN J. SMITH is a writer from the Newport Writers for Recovery Workshop.

GEORGE THOMAS, a former French horn player, grew up in Connecticut and has done radio shows for 40 years. George is one of the 2,000 people who goes out and buys a new book of poetry on a regular basis. An avid photographer, he is trying to write to understand how words, music, and images fit into a sober life.

KURTIS THOMPSON is a native Vermonter who grew up on a dirt road in the middle of nowhere. Ever since he was five years old he has wanted to be a writer. His older sister was the champion of getting him sober, however not long after he did so, she was beaten into a coma and died four months later. Kurtis is currently going to school in hope of becoming a high school English and/or history teacher.

CAROL VAN ETTEN is a writer from the Barre Writers for Recovery Workshop.

STAN WORTHLEY is a recovering addict and alcoholic who has lived with PTSD for 30 years and self-medicated for 20 years. His recovery was only able to begin after he started writing about his experiences.

Writers for Recovery is generously supported by the following organizations and individuals:

THE RONA JAFFE FOUNDATION

THE VERMONT DEPARTMENT OF CORRECTIONS

BURLINGTON LABS

THE VERMONT ASSOCIATION OF MENTAL HEALTH AND
ADDICTION RECOVERY/ PEAR-VT

THE BEN AND JERRY'S FOUNDATION

BARI AND PETER DREISSIGACKER

THE VERMONT ARTS COUNCIL

FOULKES DESIGN

EPIPHANY MAGAZINE

WILLARD COOK

SYDNEY LEA

JOHN ROSENBLUM

SUSAN RITZ

NAT AND MARTHA WINTHROP

GEOFFREY KANE